CHRONIC DISEASE

A WORKING HYPOTHESIS

※

BY
E. BACH, M.B., B.S., D.P.H.
AND
C. E. WHEELER, M.D., B.S., B.Sc.

※

British Library Cataloguing-in-Publication Data
A catalogue record for this book is available from
the British Library

AUTHORS' PREFACE.

We wish most gratefully to acknowledge the kindness of several physicians, to whom we are deeply indebted. They have not only given us permission to use cases wherein we have had the honour to co-operate with them in treatment, but have also supplied us with the necessary details of their histories. We are under a special debt of gratitude to :—

Dr. Moore of Eastbourne, Dr. Hewer and Dr. Wells of Stratford-on-Avon.

Our thanks are also due to the Otto Beit Research Fund and to the Committee which directs its use, for grants made in aid of the work of daily bacteriological investigation of a number of cases, sufficient to enable us to trace the rise and fall in bacterial out-put which is described in Chapter 3, and to Dr. A. Macgowan for help given to us in this work.

CONTENTS.

CHRONIC DISEASE

A WORKING HYPOTHESIS

INTRODUCTION

IT is doubtful if any short period in the history of medicine has been more productive of new knowledge and consequently of new conceptions than the last twenty years. If it were possible to detach problems of disease and recovery from individual needs and consider them in the abstract, it might well be that the medical profession would be slower to attempt to deduce methods of treatment from their experiences and would delay until prolonged experiment and observation had removed some of the empiricism which now, necessarily, attaches to efforts to make use of the new knowledge in daily practice.

But obviously this is impossible. The Public Health Official is free from the individual patient in his work of prevention of disease, but the practitioner, general or consultant, is regarded as the vendor of cure or at least of relief to the sufferer, who may be forgiven if he thinks that there is nothing else in the world so important as the disappearance of his particular pain and discomfort. If the regular profession fail him (or her), there are always the patent medicine vendors clutching greedily at any scrap of knowledge that can be pressed into the service of their advertisements and the enthusiastic proclaimers of any number of panaceas from spinal manipulations to Christian Science formulas.

Consequently whenever physicians see, even dimly, facts new and old grouping themselves in a more orderly manner and suggesting new conceptions of life and its variations of health and of disease, they would be less than human if they did not try to turn their vision to practical account in the treatment of patients. We know that at best much of our knowledge can be no more than an approximation to the truth to be superseded in its turn, but we must use our vision as far as it extends. If the satirists from Molière to Bernard Shaw and Jules Romains deride us that we dogmatize over-much and boast of our clearness of eyesight beyond the measure, we may at least plead that it is our own patient work (not that of the scoffer) which sifts the few grains of wheat from the masses of chaff and toil-somely harvests them. Also we have in some sort learnt their lesson and take their derision (in the words of one of them) less as an insult than as a tonic.

The problems of chronic disease have been greatly illumined by the realization of the frequency and gravity of local infections. Bacteriology can suggest remedies for those that can be discovered. Of late the bowel, particularly the colon, has been singled out for reprobation to such an extent, that the words Intestinal Toxaemia form almost too convenient a diagnosis for obscure disease conditions, and the scientifically minded are almost tempted to despair over a name that seems to recall the phrases of our great-grandfathers in its vagueness and universality.

Nevertheless that the bowel *is* the source of a variety of poisons, that their absorption into the system *is* the cause of much illness may be regarded as beyond doubt. It is the purpose of this book to attempt to trace at least one group of intestinal poisons to their source and suggest a treatment for them. In other words we believe that in many cases we can substitute for the vague diagnosis of Intestinal Toxaemia a precise statement as to the dietetic errors which permit definite bacteria to thrive and suggest means (bacteriological and dietetic) to deal with the whole condition. Our conclusions are based on ten year's work, bacteriological and clinical, and our results are such that we desire to invite as wide a testing as possible of both conclusions and practice. For if our colleagues can confirm us out of their experience they will find themselves possessed of a new and powerful weapon for the treatment of chronic disease and if they cannot confirm us, then one more hopeful path will be shown to be a blind alley and we can all turn to new explorations.

We propose to adopt the following plan in our exposition of our beliefs and methods. First to consider the state of the bowel contents as they generally are and as they might be. Then to discuss the causes of the customary state which we regard as poisonous even when actual obvious disease symptoms are few or slight. Finally, to discuss by what means the state of the bowel contents can be modified. We have to consider Diet, Bacteriology, and Vaccine treatment, and perhaps it will be best first to state our case as a thesis and proceed thereafter to examine it in detail. The thesis consists of a study of some of the existing facts, of deductions from them as to their possible causes and of the clinical results obtained by acting on these deductions. Briefly it may be stated thus :—

The ordinary diet of civilized life predisposes to chronic bacterial infections of the intestinal tract. These infections vary in their virulence but the essential factor which makes them dangerous is their chronicity. Single doses of their toxins by tests on animals may appear but slightly virulent (if at all), but the cumulative effect of them absorbed day in and day out, year after year, is a potent cause of many varieties of chronic disease.

We speak of " toxins " of the bacteria, but if further investigations reveal that the essential poisons are derived from the food taken, we shall be of opinion that these poisonous food derivatives are the result of the bacterial growth. So that to check the latter will diminish the amount of the former. That for instance Indol and Skatol are poisonous is easily enough shown on any individual who is bold enough to swallow them. Even a small dose, if frequently repeated, will produce long lasting and unpleasant results. Moreover, Skatol and Indol are end products and (like most end products) probably much less toxic than their precursors. The causes of certain chronic diseases may be indeed two-fold, bacterial toxins and food derivatives, the bye product of bacterial metabolism. To check the growth of the bacteria lessens both kinds of poison.

It is very doubtful whether, when once firmly established, any change of diet will remove these bacteria entirely, although suitable dieting is of great (sometimes of vital) importance. But although natural specific resistance to these infections is but imperfectly developed, the process can be notably influenced by vaccines appropriate to the case and administered in the appropriate manner. The clinical results of vaccine treatment, whereof over ten years we have a large number, both tend to confirm the view that the infections are related causally to the diseases and to confirm the hopefulness of this means of dealing with them. These results will be summarized later as they form an important part of our case.

Before, however, we proceed to examine this thesis in detail we must guard against one misconception. Although there are good bacteriologists who dismiss, as non-toxic, strains of bacteria which we regard as among the direst enemies of mankind, there are many besides ourselves, pathologists and clinicians, who agree with us so far at least. The last thing which we wish to imply is that we are the only or the most important workers in this field. Far from it. Our claim to speak is founded on two considerations. First, we believe that our actual method of administering vaccines in these cases is of such importance that success may entirely depend upon it. Secondly, this opinion is backed by a longer clinical experience than has fallen to the lot of many. We ask no more than to be regarded as explorers of a province of medicine which many others have worked over, without perhaps happening on our particular treasures. These we offer to the common stock of medical knowledge to be tested, whether they be true gold or worthless metal.

CHAPTER I

DIET AND ITS DISABILITIES.

IT is not our purpose to enter in detail into the physiology of digestion but rather to emphasize a few of its ordinary phenomena and draw, if we may, a few conclusions from them. Our observations do not contradict accepted doctrine although their importance is not always fully realized.

Most men and women, in the absence of symptoms of abdominal pain or discomfort, are satisfied with a regular daily action of the bowels, even sometimes with an action on every alternate day. The vast quantities of purgative patent medicines consumed tend to show that this result is not achieved without some assistance, but such as it is it is the commonly accepted standard for persons living on the ordinary mixed diet of civilized (western) countries. The ordinary stool, thus, as it were, standardized, varies from hard masses to soft even semi-solid material but with hardly an exception in adult life it is more or less dark, foul smelling and alkaline in reaction. Alkaline also is the reaction of the large bowel from which it proceeds. If an emulsion of a small portion is made and cultures taken, bacteria will grow freely, Coli and Streptococci and spore-bearing organisms always, and almost invariably bacilli of the non-lactose-fermenting group. The detailed bacteriology will be dealt with in the next chapter, at the moment we are more concerned with the grosser factors of which the foulness and the alkalinity are the most important. The alkalinity favours notably the growth of certain strains of organisms and the compounds that cause the foulness are notoriously poisonous if absorbed in any quantity into the blood, a phenomenon favoured by the bowel stasis and retention of faeces which so often occurs, since one of the commonest poisonous effects is a deadening of reflexes and an inertia of muscle response. Constipation is directly encouraged and a vicious circle of phenomena easily established. Now if an ordinary man or woman, in so-called ordinary health, will live for some weeks on a special diet, changes will ensue in the appearance and general character of the faeces. The diet must be of food as largely as possible uncooked. Raw fruit with good quantities of nuts (well masticated), vegetables, salads, dairy produce, wholemeal bread, cereals, milk puddings : and for fluids, water, weak tea, milk : wines of all kinds are permissible but not spirits. —After a variable time, covering in any case some weeks and often running to months,* the character of the faeces will change. They will become bright yellow, soft, semi-solid, entirely

*The time needed can be shortened by a preliminary fast of some days.

odourless and acid in reaction. Actions may become almost embarrassingly frequent, for peristalsis (though free from any painful sensations, and unaccompanied by gross fermentation and flatulence) is readily encouraged and any food taken into the stomach is apt to initiate muscular bowel movements that end in defaecation. Bacteriologically there is a great diminution in all organisms that thrive in an alkaline medium, namely, B. Coli, Streptococci and spore-bearing bacilli. Of the utmost importance is the appearance of the Lactic acid bacillus, virtually non-existent in the alkaline stools, but multiplying in response to this diet until it may constitute as much as 30 per cent. of the total bacterial flora. If the individual has habitually eaten much meat or otherwise departed far from this special diet in ordinary life, or is heavily infected with the non-lactose-fermenting bacilli, he (or she) may take a long time to effect these changes in faecal characteristics and may never exactly reproduce those described. But whoever will faithfully follow the diet will achieve them in a greater rather than in a lesser degree.

If these acid fæces are distilled—and the absence of stinking compounds makes this quite feasible in an ordinary laboratory —a volatile fatty acid comes over freely. Such investigations as have been made, indicate that the acid is not one of the better known members of the series. Further work is in progress as to this point. Here it suffices to say that its presence is of vital importance to the bacteriology of the lower bowel. The strains of organisms whose growth it hinders are precisely those whose presence we regard as harmful in a high degree. It is therefore not surprising that there should usually be an increased sense of well-being in those who persist in this diet, marked even among persons who do not regard themselves as being unwell and more marked in many chronic sufferers. Sleep becomes more restful and less of it is required, energy increases, sense of fatigue diminishes.

So far these results, doubtless familiar to physicians, tend to confirm the general theories of intestinal toxæmia. If the toxæmias are due to bacterial products the acid bowel checks their growth and thus toxæmia lessens. If the chronic poisoning is the result of absorption of decomposition products from food, the result of stasis, then, stasis being modified and decomposition products being absent, the system is relieved. If both factors are at work, both are being dealt with and the improved health seems a natural consequence. Surely it is only reasonable to believe that it is less desirable to have the lower bowel continually filled with its usual foul contents than with the odour'ess fæces which are the consequence of a suitable diet, even apart from specific bacterial infections. It seems obvious that there must be less toxic material to be absorbed in the latter case. But more remains to be said.

First be it noted that in the dietary outlined above stress is laid on uncooked food. Many vegetarians eat actually little more raw food than the ordinary citizen and thereby probably improve but little on the ordinary citizen's habits. They may indeed deprive themselves of energy producing food-stuff without any counter-balancing gain. The true substitutes for meat in the vegetarian dietary are nuts, cereals, and possibly bananas. If these are omitted, the vegetarian is in a worse position than the meat-eater. Moreover, it is quite possible that meat and fish are much more harmful when cooked : the carnivora are not longlived but healthy enough during their span of life. The part played by food preservatives is much under discussion at the moment. It cannot conceivably be a beneficial one. Further, something seems to be lost by the freezing of meat, though

it is difficult now to picture our civilization
without cold storage   Those, therefore, who
wish to acquire an acid large intes ine and its
advantages must lay stress on the uncooked
elements in their dietary.   Particularly important in this respect is the uncooked nut
and cereal, which reaches the lower bowel
(as is well known, of course) largely as
starch and hydrolysing there supplies food
for the B. Lacticus, who has a poor time of
it in the colon of the average citizen.   To
swallow cultures of the Bacillus and then to
starve it seems unreasonable.   Failure to
realize its need of nourishment goes far to
explain the many disappointments of the
Sour Milk treatments.   It follows further
that the addition of raw nut and cereal
alone to an ordinary diet may (and often
does) do a great deal of good in altering
the character of the stool and the condition of the large intestine.

However, before we can expect civilized
races thus drastically to reconsider their

diet they will require more assurance
as to the rewards which they may expect.
They will ask : will they acquire an intestinal
tract free of all pathogenic bacteria ? The
answer is almost certainly in the negative.
A suitable diet will reduce pathogenic
bacteria in numbers and (perhaps) in virulence and food-decomposition products will
disappear, but in our judgement a tract once
thoroughly infected is seldom, if ever,
cleared by diet alone : some anti-bacterial
measures are needed in addition. These
will be considered presently and thereafter
it may be possible to pronounce on the
relative importance of diet and vaccines.
Assuredly they supplement one another,
but we have to grasp some more facts before
we are in a position to form satisfactory
conclusions. This chapter states the altera-
tions that can be achieved in the bowel and
its contents by Diet alone. It is now time
to turn to the Bacteriology of the Fæces.

Dr. Chetam Strode's advocacy of raw oatmeal is well-known
("Simple means of lessening or eliminating alimentary Toxæmia,
Lancet, 1920"). Oatmeal being the richest food stuff known in
starch, a smaller quantity of it is required to supply the B. Lacticus
with its necessary food than of other cereals. The addition of not
less than 3 to 4 ounces daily to an ordinary dietary often suffices to
produce beneficial changes.

CHAPTER II

THE BACTERIAL CONTENT OF THE FAECES

THE bacterial content of fæces, such as are found in civilised countries and usually regarded as normal, is undoubtedly very far removed from the true normal and one of the most striking effects of the cleansing of the intestine is the great change in its bacterial flora ; purgatives, intestinal antiseptics and ordinary therapeutic measures have little permanent effect and do not cause any marked alteration in this respect.

Suitable diet, certainly, may alter the picture, but if there is a profound infection of long standing even a strict diet may need many months before it produces any definite result.

The abnormal organisms, which so much interfere with the complete cleansing of the gut, probably have their stronghold in the gall bladder, where antiseptics are unable to reach them (*cf.* typhoid carriers), and in the present state of knowledge the vaccine alone appears able to eradicate these invaders with any degree of success.

The organisms usually found in civilisation are the following :—

Bacillus Coli.
Streptococci.
Spore-bearing bacilli.
Other Gram-negative bacilli.

The bacilli found in clean fæces are :—

Bacillus Coli.
Lactic Acid Bacillus.

The Bacillus Coli. This organism is in all probability a normal inhabitant, as it is found not only in man under all conditions but also in animals and birds.

Streptococci are more difficult to place as normal or abnormal organisms : they are almost as commonly present in man as the

B. Coli and in animals to a certain extent although in cases where the intestines have been thoroughly cleansed they may disappear.

Spore-bearing Bacilli, the group of which Bacillus Welchii and Tetanus are members, are found generally both in man and animals, but they disappear entirely in the human properly treated.

The Lactic Acid Bacillus is found in carnivora and herbivora and in man when eating sufficient raw material. Apparently it is unable to thrive without the presence of sugar or starch in the large gut ; it is the organism which produces the acid of the cæcum and is a Gram-positive bacillus without spores, growing anærobically. By changing the diet the percentage of this bacillus in the fæcal flora may be made to change enormously in a few days.

The other *Gram-negative Organisms* have been left to the last because it is necessary to lay stress upon them. They are members of the great group known as the *Coli-Typhoid*. (We exclude here those that are of definite pathological virulence, such as Typhoid, the varieties of Dysentery and Paratyphoids.) Their number is probably almost without limit, though most of them can be placed into one of the subclasses of the main group. Many of them have been named, but such is their variety that it is possible to examine forty or fifty without finding two identical. It is rather the rule for bacteriologists to dismiss many of these bacilli as non-pathogenic, but a point which we particularly wish to stress is that a non-lactose-fermenting Gram-negative bacillus in the fæces, whether it falls into a known variety or not, may be the cause of toxæmia, even though it may not give rise to obvious lesions. In fact the great majority probably never do, nor can, cause locally anything more than at the most, a little mucous colitis or some affection of that nature.

These organisms are readily obtained by

plating the fæces on ordinary media ;
McKonki's bile salt, lactose, neutral red,
peptone agar being used in our work. *See
Appendix B.* It is extraordinary how
frequently only one examination is necessary
to find a non-lactose fermenter, but in some
cases more than one examination is required,
and more rarely many platings before the
desired result is obtained ; but if patience
is exercised and sufficient specimens exa-
mined, it will be found in virtually one
hundred per cent. of cases that an abnormal
bacillus of this type will ultimately be
found. In the few instances which give
negative results persistently, a dose of a
polyvalent vaccine will usually cause a large
percentage of the patient's own organism
to appear within a few days.

The fundamental characteristic of these
bacilli is that they are members of the Coli-
Typhoid group, which do not ferment lactose.
As their varieties are unending it is not
possible, conveniently, to attempt to name

such as may be isolated, but only to relegate them to groups, according to their sugar reactions. There is still a wide field for research in this direction, because from the limited observations we have made, there is reason to believe that the symptoms caused depend in some measure on the type of bacillus present in the patient and further work may narrow this down to a very considerable extent. The great majority of organisms obtained ferment glucose, giving acid and gas and do not ferment lactose or saccharose.

In addition to members of the Coli-Typhoid group, bacilli of the Proteus type may be found now and then, most frequently in epilepsy, stammering, and varieties of recurring " nerve storm."

Another group which may occasionally occur is the Pyocyaneus type, although this is generally associated with obvious lesions. Abnormal organisms of such types may be found at all ages and we have frequently obtained them in infants of a few months old, probably infected from cow milk which contains them, or from the nipple or hands of a parent. So common are these bacilli that the question may be raised, are they not normal inhabitants ? The reasons for a negative answer are twofold, first the extraordinary benefit obtained with vaccines of them in chronic disease ; and next their disappearance in patients so treated.

These organisms interfere with the action of the Lactic Acid Bacilli in their production of acid and it is for this reason that diet of raw material is not alone able to produce a clean intestine in the more severe cases. It is common in a patient who has dieted regularly for some time with little or no benefit, to obtain almost at once an acid reaction and improve symptomatically after an inoculation of vaccine.

The acid reaction of the large intestine is of importance in two ways ; first it inhibits the growth of these bacilli and secondly it supplies an acid medium in which (as is common knowledge in every laboratory), bacteria are not able to produce toxins to any extent comparable to their ability to do so in an alkaline medium. It is for this reason that in practice it is usual to add an alkaline salt to broth in which toxins are being prepared, to neutralise any acid formed and thus allow the organisms, diphtheria or whatever they may be, full scope.

Moreover, fermentation as it occurs in the large intestine is altogether different under alkaline and under acid conditions, and apart from bacterial toxins many of the more dangerous poisons obtainable from protein are not formed in an acid medium.

The particular object of this chapter is to emphasise the universality in civilisation of these non-lactose-fermenting bacilli and to suggest that they are capable of producing toxins harmful to the individual and interfering with the natural cleansing organisms of the intestine, the Lactic Acid Bacilli.

CHAPTER III.

THE NATURE AND TREATMENT OF CHRONIC DISEASE.

THE foregoing chapters set together the more obvious facts with regard to the effect of diet (ordinary and special) on intestinal contents and on the bacteriology of the bowel. From them it is apparent that the usual diet of civilized Western Life results in the development of excess of poisonous substances and of a very free bacterial flora wherein non-Gram, non-lactose-fermenting organisms can be almost invariably isolated. But while these fæcal characteristics and bacterial flora are found in most cases of chronic disease (even of most diverse types and symtomatology), they can also be discovered, if sought for, in subjects who make no complaint of illness and maintain that they are in perfect health.

Clearly therefore there is yet another

factor to be reckoned with before obvious
illness results from these unhealthy bowel
conditions. That factor is probably the
relative permeability of the bowel wall.
There can be little doubt that a healthy
intestinal wall resists the passage both of
bacterial toxins and poisonous food derivatives. Provided that the wall is a genuine
barrier quite a high degree of stasis is
compatible with the absence of disease
symptoms, although peristaltic inertia should
itself be regarded as a sign (usually the first
sign) of absorption of poison and will in-
fallibly, sooner or later, prove the precursor
of graver troubles. But all physicians are
familiar with the cases that occur every now
and then, wherein for years of apparent
health the lower bowel has to be evacuated
by enema once a week or even once a fort-
night. Further, it is often observed that
the constipated who suffer also from such
symptoms as headache, lassitude and weari-
ness, are more likely so to suffer during

purgation (the " enema rash " is a similar phenomenon), because the presence of more fluid in the bowel no doubt encourages toxic absorption. They actually absorb less and consequently feel better during the constipated periods. This obviously does not mean that constipation is a desirable state, but it does imply that merely to ensure some sort of daily action of the bowels is not in itself sufficient to guarantee a healthy tract. Many sufferers from alimentary toxæmia can (and do) boast of a daily action of the bowels and are by no means inclined to believe that nevertheless the tract may be unhealthy.

Relative permeability of the bowel wall to toxins or other poisons is therefore the factor which decides whether unnatural diet and consequent (for it is in the main consequent) morbid bacterial growths will result in disease or no. Or perhaps it would be more exact to say that it is relative permeability which decides *when* the morbid bowel phenomena will result in obvious symptoms of disease.

It is more than likely that permeability of the bowel wall varies widely in different subjects. It may well be a characteristic that is inherited and the tendency of certain diseases to " run in families," the inheritance of a " diathesis " in the sense in which French physicians used to employ the term, may ultimately be referable to a greater or less bowel permeability. Be this as future investigation may determine, it is surely reasonable to believe that in general the bowel starts life well and maintains its health in youth and early life better than later, for there is no bodily function which does not find the stresses of civilized life and the burden of advancing years to be factors which weaken and impede. Life's reserves tend to be spent and the time comes for us all when they are less available.

If therefore, faulty diet and morbid bacterial growths are common to most of the population, a greater or less permeability of the bowel and especially a permeability tending to increase as life advances would account for the fact that the morbid phenomena of Chronic disease (apart from such well defined disorders as Venereal Disease and Tuberculosis), tend to appear increasingly as youth passes into middle age and as middle age advances. But it does not follow that the young who show few or no symptoms are therefore to be regarded as healthy. On the contrary our contention is that, given an unhealthy bowel content, some kind of chronic disease is certain to occur sooner or later and that the surest way to ward it off is to get the bowel physiologically clean and maintain it so. We believe the sequence of events to be as follows :—ordinary diet, owing to its insufficiency in natural carbo-hydrates, is unable to cause the lactic acid bacilli to thrive in the large intestine, and the reaction of the contents of the gut remain alkaline.

In this alkaline medium proteolytic bacteria thrive and produce probably not only their own toxins but also harmful derivatives from the food ; which, when their application is continued over a long period of time may cause an increased permeability of the mucous membrane ; thus allowing poisons to be more readily absorbed and the organisms to become established in the gut wall.

We believe that, if from birth the content of the intestine was normal, abnormal organisms would have the greatest difficulty of infecting the bowel wall. Even after bacterial toxins and poisonous food derivatives begin to pass through, as their grade of toxicity is not very high symptoms may be few and slight, but the action is cumulative because the production is constant and morbid phenomena sooner or later appear too obviously to be missed. The man or woman is now a patient and seeks medical aid for an illness that appears to the sufferer of recent origin, but has in actual fact been latent and developing for years.

This is the essence of our conception of the origin and development of many chronic diseases and the explanation of the undoubted fact that the factors of diet and bowel conditions which we regard as morbid, exist in early life, yet cause in the majority of cases no obvious symptoms. We regard the factor of time as essential in the production of chronic disease. In other words we conceive a poison of slight immediate virulence as capable of developing disease by dint of its persistence.

But it will justly be contended here, " By what right do you regard these organisms as causal ? By your own confession they are often present without symptoms of disease, indeed, you have to invoke a special explanation to get over that fact and assume a greater or less permeability of the bowel which cannot be directly demonstrated. You must relate the organisms to disease more directly than you have so far done, before there can be question of conceding you anything of that sort." This is a fair demand and it must be met.

The reasons for regarding these Gram-negative, non-lactose-fermenting organisms as the causes of chronic disease are almost entirely clinical. Since the organisms require a very long time of slow poisoning before symptoms of disease appear, the reproduction of the diseases in animals would be difficult. It would be first necessary so to modify the animals' diet that the organisms could thrive in the bowel. The rabbit or guinea pig on an ordinary diet will not tolerate them. But the principles of vaccine therapy are by this time sufficiently established to warrant the belief that if disease symptoms disappear or are much ameliorated after the use of a vaccine made from a particular organism or organisms, then that (or those) organisms count at least for something in the production of the disease symptoms. One of the great features of modern medicine is the search for focal infections and, provided an organism is found, the advisability of trying a vaccine made from it, would be generally conceded by all, at any rate, except by the few who reject entirely the belief that germs have anything to do with disease.

Our main reason for believing that these organisms are the causes of disease rests on the very striking curative results obtained by using vaccines made from them. Details will be given in the next two chapters, but it may be stated here, that if in cases of chronic disease intestinal organisms are found, then vaccines made from them will produce swift and striking results in at least 15 per cent, excellent though more gradual results in another 65 per cent. and some definite response in another 15 per cent, leaving only about 5 per cent. un- affected. One proviso must, however, be made. The results will not be obtained unless the technique of administration is faithfully followed. There will be more to say of this presently ; at the moment it is enough to state that it consists essentially in allowing each dose time to develop a favourable reaction and not repeating an injection as long as improvement continues, even though the period of waiting lasts for weeks or months.

Provided then that the vaccines are suitably used, their results are so striking that it is very difficult to resist the conviction that the organisms are related to the disease as cause and effect. But the clinical results can be supported by some interesting direct observations.

When these Gram-negative, non-lactose-fermenting organisms are carefully looked for, they are usually readily found.* Sometimes repeated examinations are necessary, however, and occasionally the organisms are persistently absent, even when

*(Appendix B gives details of the cultural technique employed).

symptoms strongly suggest that they are
present and active. When we had convinced ourselves that these organisms were
genuine causes of disease, it was natural to
try the effect of a stock vaccine on cases
wherein they could not be found, although their disease symptoms were similar
to those met with in undoubted chronic
infections with bacteria of this type. The
results were almost invariably striking. Not
only did the cases respond and the symptoms improve, but organisms of the now
familiar type began to appear freely in the
fæces, exactly as though they were being
thrown off from the bowel as a result of the
favourable response to the stock vaccine.
This observation (repeated in a number of
separate cases), led to further investigations.

In a number of cases wherein organisms
had been found and autogenous vaccines
were being used, examinations were made
of every stool passed for weeks together
and the following phenomena were always

observed *for every case that improved, i.e.,
responded to the vaccine.* If the percentage
of suspected organisms to the total bacterial
flora were (say) 5 per cent. before the vaccine was given (this is quite a typical
number), then immediately after the vaccine
the percentage would diminish or even
disappear. This drop in numbers corres-
ponds to the period of reaction during
which the patient usually feels definitely
worse, often with gastro-intestinal symptoms. In favourable cases, this period of
aggravation of symptoms seldom lasts long.
If it endures for more than a week, that is
usually an indication that the initial dose
was too large and great care and patience
will be needed to handle the case successfully.
In most cases, fortunately, improvement
soon sets in. At once the organisms reappear in the stools and quickly the percentage of them rises. The 5 per cent.
becomes, 10, 20, 50 per cent. and may go
on until virtually a pure culture is obtained.

Correspondingly, in exact ratio, the patient's symptoms improve.

When presently improvement ceases the time has come for a repetition of the dose and usually a somewhat larger one is given. Reaction is seldom as severe as after the first dose ; in many cases a new spurt of improvement follows and so the case is gradually carried to recovery. In cases wherein symptoms have been present for years the maximum of recovery often demands a long time. A good (rough) estimate is to take a month of treatment for every year during which disease symptoms have persisted

The organisms will be found in large numbers during all the earlier months of treatment : but as recovery comes nearer they begin again to diminish in numbers until finally they are few or all but non-existent. Once this result is obtained, a certain care in diet and a very occasional vaccine, if any old symptoms reappear, are all that is required.

Now this parallel variation in the numbers of organisms present with the improvement in the patient, combined with the symptomatic favourable response to the vaccine, makes it doubly difficult to doubt that, between disease and organisms there is a real relation and that relation one of cause and effect. At any rate, it is upon these twin phenomena that we base our belief and if the results which we have seen are equally obtained by others the belief will become a virtual certainty. But if the likelihood is conceded that these organisms are the causes of much chronic disease, then their presence in youth (and occasionally in middle life), without disease symptoms is, nevertheless, significant. The absence of symptoms can be explained by invoking a relative non-permeability of the bowel wall but, in view of the dangers hanging over the years to come, treatment should surely be adopted even though no disease symptoms are obvious. By watching the stools bacteriologically some light may be gained as to the response to the vaccine.* Naturally, the proof that to treat these bowel infections in early life in the absence of symptoms, wards off chronic disease later, will only be forthcoming when experiments have been conducted on a very wide scale indeed. But at least it can do no harm to try and in time, out of a vast multitude of experiments, some convictions may result.

A further reason for these experiments may be suggested. We venture here into a largely untrodden land. Observations of ours, made during a dozen years, suggest certain conclusions which may be regarded as possible paths into this uncharted territory. Much more observation and experiment is needed in order to determine which are true paths and which delusive

*This involves periodical counting of the calonies obtained by plating a specimen. But even if no obvious disease symptoms are present there should be a greater sense of well-being as treatment proceeds.

ones. It is in the hope of stimulating the experiments that we put forward these suggestions. They are all based on clinical observations and on the results of the use of vaccines.

All the organisms on which we have been concentrating attention are of a low grade of virulence. They do not cause local inflammation or violent reaction. It is for this reason that they are so often regarded as non-pathogenic. But since virulent organisms are also those which quickly rouse body resistance (so that there is a swift struggle for mastery and either the body succumbs or the germ is effectively resisted and a certain protection acquired against it), so organisms not obviously virulent in all probability arouse but feeble protective responses. The system invaded is tolerant of them ; whatever toxins result from their presence are not of sufficient power or quantity to threaten life directly and for a long period there may be little or no sign that they are harmful.*

Nevertheless, the final appearance of obvious disease symptoms curable by an attack on these organisms, suggests forcibly (as has been already argued) that there is a certain slight poisoning throughout the earlier (apparently healthy) years, whose immediate slightness is overweighted by its persistence and cumulative action. The body invaded by these bacteria is *not* healthy though it may appear to be.

It is therefore of great importance to try to detect any signs of the harmful presence of these organisms even when the harm is relatively slight. Observation of a large number of established cases of chronic disease and particularly a careful record and correlation of the earliest symptoms manifested, suggest that the first harmful effects of these bacteria are exerted against the endocrine glands and that some dis-

*(Symptoms of disease are usually quite as much evidence of body reaction as of disease attack. A symptom-complex is made up of both elements in varying proportions).

turbance in endocrine balance is almost
inevitable. In the group of neurasthenias
for instance (cases in which, almost without
exception, investigations reveal the presence
of organisms of this type) a lowered blood
pressure is virtually invariable at first.
But among the functions of a normal endocrine balance resistance to ordinary germs
of local suppuration and catarrh ranks
high and this power is apt to lessen if
endocrine balance is disturbed. Consequently a lowered resistance to the commoner
pathogenic organisms, the streptococci
and staphylococci, m. catarrhalis and pneu-
mococci, etc., may be really dependent on an
underlying poisoning from intestinal organisms. The effects may appear in chronic
or frequently repeated catarrhs, in pyorrhæa
or crops of boils or whatever. The local
manifestations may vary with the special
local susceptibility and site of invasion.
Resistance to organisms appears to be made
up of factors of general resistance and

specific resistance. The suggestion made is that intestinal poisoning affects the factor of general (non-specific) resistance and that the specific resistances are insufficient to produce speedy recovery when the " general " factor is impaired. The object of vaccine therapy is to enhance resistance powers. When chronic catarrhs and other focal affections are present, autogenous vaccines (or stock vaccines) made from the focal organisms are often brilliantly successful. Nevertheless quite frequently they fail. If, when failure occurs, search is made for intestinal organisms, then if they are discovered, combined vaccines (fæcal and local) will far more often succeed than local alone. More than this, a fæcal vaccine alone will often put an end to local troubles, suggesting that the resistance factors controlled by the fæcal toxins are the more important and that if they are raised in value the greater part of the work of cure is thereby accomplished.

Even with chronic diseases the use of

vaccines made from focal infections (e.g., pyorrhæa) is seldom so successful as to warrant the belief that the focal disease is the *whole* of the evil. Sir Arbuthnot Lane and his colleagues have already maintained that intestinal toxæmia predisposes to pyorrhæa and the use of such vaccines as we are here advocating is, to say the least, a most valuable aid in clearing up both the pyorrhæa and the arthritis or whatever, which may be held to be dependent on it. We are not, for a moment, maintaining that the local infections do not require to be taken into account in treatment. Our convictions may be phrased thus :—Chronic intestinal toxæmia, from the non-lactose-fermenting organisms, lowers general bacterial resistance (possibly through its effect on endocrine secretion balance) ; consequently local bacterial infections are almost certain to occur. These add their quota to the ill-health of the patient and are not well combated because the lowered general resistance, which made their growth possible, persists. Vaccines made from the local infections may deal with them satisfactorily but more often leave much to be desired. Vaccines from the intestinal germs alone, by improving general resistance, may incidentally relieve the local infections. But the best method is to use a mixed vaccine, intestinal and local and so deal with all the factors of ill-health simultaneously. The results of this two-fold vaccination will be found most satisfactory. It should always be thought of when the focal vaccines fail.

The predisposition to other diseases which results from the presence of chronic intestinal infections may well be of importance with regard to more deadly diseases—e.g., Tuberculosis and Rheumatism. The classical dyspepsia of early Phthisis is held to be a symptom of actual Tuberculosis, but it is not without significance from the point of view of possible intestinal toxæmia. At any rate the intestinal organisms are usually found in Tuberculosis if sought for ; but considerable caution is needed in the use of intestinal vaccines in this disease. A dose, unless very small, is very liable to cause a severe aggravation of the Tubercular symptoms and cases of latent Tubercle may be roused to activity by an incautious administration of an intestinal vaccine. These unfavourable results certainly suggest that the intestinal poisons play a predisposing part in the causation of Tuberculosis, so marked that the " negative phase " which follows the vaccine administration becomes a period of definite danger. Consequently, only the very smallest doses must be given and these with caution and all the factors of sunlight and air and suitable food, which enhance general resistance, should be fully employed at the same time. Not, of course, that these general factors should ever be neglected but in Tuberculosis they are, if possible, more urgent than ever.*

*Specialists in Tuberculosis are coming increasingly to believe that symptoms of active Tubercular disease occurring in adolescence or later are traceable to primary infections acquired in early life remaining, for the most part, quiescent until some extra stress encourages them to develop. If this opinion proves correct we suggest that the factor of Chronic Intestinal poisoning may frequently constitute the actual extra stress that determines the attack of obvious Tuberculosis.

It is in our experience quite possible to have Tuberculosis arrested and yet to have chronic intestinal toxæmia remaining. This shows that, however the latter may predispose to Tuberculosis, the resistance to Tubercle can function independently. But these cases are by no means well although their Tuberculosis is in abeyance and the treatment of them by intestinal vaccines, with due caution against the danger of reviving latent Tubercle, is satisfactory in the end though usually very slow.

Patience in fact, as has already been stated, is essential for the proper treatment of these diseases. The sufferer's choice is between seeking relief for the time of exacerbation of symptoms (asthma paroxysms, acute or subacute arthritis, recurrent psoriasis or eczema or whatever), and " carrying on " more or less satisfactorily in the intervals : or of seeking a cure as permanent as may be by systematic treatment over a considerable time. As will be

presently pointed out the latter need not
(does not) mean a great deal of either time
or money spent on the physician : but it
does mean a regular course of treatment
checked and guided by regular reports.
If the patient prefers the method of relief
of severe symptoms only he will suffer
increasingly as the years advance until a
real cure becomes impossible because
permanent damage has been done to non-
replaceable tissues.*   But if patient and
physician seek for cure then time must
be given to achieve it.

The essence of the whole matter is that
our bodies do not react strongly against
these organisms but tolerate them far too
readily.   In other words whatever anti-
bodies we are capable of manufacturing
against them are neither present normally
nor readily prepared. The business of
resistance is a delicate one, a plant of tender
growth, easily checked and nurtured with

*Not always in the same way : skin diseases may alternate with,
or replace arthritis or *vice versa*, or new symptoms may appear.

difficulty. The organisms may be likened to those hordes of aliens who loom in the dreams of some timorous patriots : insidous invaders too easily tolerated by a trustful nation preparing the direst disasters for future years. But while the patriots seek to meet their danger by shouting and clamour, far more subtle measures are needed for the body's invaders. To drop metaphor, since clearness of statement is here essential, the response to vaccines in the case of these organisms is so delicate that it can only be elicited by small initial doses and long intervals between doses. Usually the first vaccine consists of two million organisms and, as has been already stated, if a favourable result follows the initial reaction, no further dose must be given for as long a time as progress is being made—whether progress be slow or rapid. More than that, since it is in the nature of all bodily processes to show a certain rhythm, progress will follow a curve, there will be good weeks and weeks

not so good. The mere occurrence of one
of the latter is not in itself an indication
for a second dose of vaccine. Only when
the case has been watched longer and it is
clear that no rise is going to follow the fall
can repetition be allowed. Now a slightly
larger dose is admissible and then patience
must again be exercised. Too much stress
cannot be laid on the need for spacing out
the doses. No real success will be obtained
unless this rule is followed.

It is in this matter, probably, that readers
will find most difficulty. While, for our
part, we are convinced that all vaccines
tend to be given too frequently and in over
large doses, it is nevertheless true that
many cases do well treated by the usual
methods. But they are not cases in which
those intestinal organisms are being used,
but gonococcal or streptococcal or pneumococcal or other secondary infections. Whenever we have tried to " push " the vaccines
of these non-lactose-fermenting bacteria,

we have only achieved failure.

Consider for a moment what we conceive ourselves to be doing when we give a vaccine : eliciting a response from the body which will be available against a particular invader. We are not attacking the invaders directly, but indirectly, trying to set in motion a machinery that has stopped or at least make more effective a machinery that is halting.

But once we realise that we are trying to influence a natural process, what is the sense of hammering away at it when once we have reason to believe that it is satisfactorily set going ? Surely then wisdom is to wait until it shows signs of flagging once more, not to assume that it must necessarily flag always after the same interval of time and fix that interval at a week or ten days. Why should not the time during which a response continues vary with the individual case ? It is much more natural to assume that it does, for that is the way of living processes, endless variability.   Broadly speaking diseases fall into a definite series in regard to their suitable vaccines.   In acute disorders (e.g., Pneumonia) the two or three doses which should be sufficient (if they are not, nothing is gained by going on) need to be given within, probably, 48 hours.   In sub-acute or markedly local diseases (" gonorrheal joints, nasal catarrhs, etc.) the suitable interval may extend to days but hardly to weeks.   But for chronic diseases the interval must be much longer and these of which we speak in this book are the most chronic of all.   It is far more easy to spoil a good case by repeating the vaccine too soon than by waiting over long.   So inert is the system, so disinclined, as it were, to take any effective measures against its insidious enemy, that it must be handled most gently and patiently and given all the time that it needs to become properly resistant.

This chapter will have raised in the

reader's mind as many queries as it will have answered. Possibly many more than it will have dealt with. But its main object is to encourage the personal experiments lacking which there can be no real conviction for or against our conclusions.

It seems best, therefore, next to give some details of actual results and that is the business of the two ensuing chapters. Thereafter will follow an attempt to indicate the most urgent lines for future investigation and incidentally give any supplementary details of treatment which bear directly on the matter in hand. Here we have argued that, since vaccine therapy in general is held to be sound practice by the great majority of the profession, the clinical results of vaccines in these classes of chronic diseases are evidence which may be adduced that the organisms indicated are the causes of the diseases. Some details of our own clinical results will show in some measure what is the extent of our evidence.

CHAPTER IV.

IT is on the clinical results which have
been obtained that our hypothesis
mainly rests and in this chapter they
are considered in detail. In all we have
taken 500 cases. Thirty-three of these are
of malignant disease and are separately
considered. The cases have not been in any
way selected, but taken from the records
(our own and those of physicians with whom
we have been associated in treatment), just
as they came ; therefore we can offer them
as a fair sample of the kind of work which
we have been doing. Two criteria we have
ins.sted on however in compiling our list.
We have omitted all cases that have not been
cbserved for at least six months and we have
omitted all cases wherein vaccines made
from intestinal germs were only part of the

total treatment. It is necessary to have a case under observation for at least six months before any valid judgement is possible as to its progress and the great majority of ours have been observed for much longer periods, so that the degree of endurance of any improvement can be fairly estimated. The only exceptions to the six months rule are some of our complete failures, wherein patients abandoned treatment either because of impatience at getting no immediate benefit or (more often) because of inability to endure a rather severe reaction. While in these cases we should much have preferred to keep in touch with the patients for six months, we have not felt justified in omitting them from our records because they tell against the final result and we are anxious not to appear to consider only successes. On the contrary we have endeavoured to give, if anything, more place relatively to our failures, feeling that this, in the present stage of our knowledge, gives the fairer basis for judgment. With regard to other methods of treatment we have not included cases wherein important accessory measures have been used. These comprise vaccines made from such septic foci as exist in pyorrhœa, chronic nasal catarrh etc., regular courses of drug or spa treatment, forms of electric treatment and so on. The most important omissions, from our point of view, are those of the cases treated by combined vaccines. We have records of two hundred to three hundred cases of chronic catarrhs (mainly respiratory), wherein a vaccine from an intestinal organism was combined with vaccine from the locality obviously affected. The results are uniformly successful, but the sceptical might readily attribute success to the catarrhal vaccine rather than to the admixture of vaccine from non-lactose-fermenting organisms. Our own belief, that the addition of the vaccine derived from the bowel organisms is the most important factor in obtaining success, is based on repeated experiences of failure of the vaccines made from the catarrhal organisms, alone, followed by cure or marked relief as soon as vaccine from the intestinal flora is added. Nevertheless, except for one or two cases wherein this sequence of failure of the partial vaccine followed by marked success of the total vaccine was very striking indeed, all these cases have been omitted from our series.

The clinical record then is made up of cases wherein any favourable results seem most reasonably attributable to vaccines made from intestinal organisms since these constituted the essential treatment. Even dieting (about which we have not hesitated to express decided opinions), was refused by nearly half the total number of patients, so that if the vaccines used are to be rejected as the prime causes of the improvement so frequently obtained, the only remaining explanation possible will be that of suggestion, of a mental influence powerful enough to produce favourable physical changes. No physician to-day is inclined to under-rate the effects of these mental influences ; but perhaps one or two comments may be allowed to us. In the first place, there is hardly a case in our series that has not tried treatments of all sorts before coming into our hands, for all are cases of chronic disease and chronic disease means as a rule, much medical advice (not to mention that of well-meaning friends), and varieties of therapeutic experiments. It is because, in the main, these have failed that the patients have come to vaccine treatment, and a series of disappointments does not create a very hopeful atmosphere or one very encouraging to the reception of suggestion. If these patients are so susceptible to mental influences that our procedure implants a curative suggestion, it is a little odd that the phenomenon did not occur earlier as a result of other (often more dramatic), therapeutic methods.

But it may be urged that our confident expectation of improvement may lead us to confident promises and that thereby a more favourable atmosphere is created for receiving suggestions. True, we are now reasonably confident that some favourable result will follow our treatment, but many of our good cases occurred in the early days when we had not had enough experience to feel more than hopeful. Further in the present state of our knowledge we have few grounds upon which to base a detailed prognosis. Some improvement we certainly expect, but whether it will be swift and dramatic, or steady and continuous, or temporary and disappointing or even absent altogether, we can seldom, if ever, prophesy with any assurance. Consequently, we are very chary indeed of bold promises for the future and the atmosphere favourable to mental influences is not (consciously at least) created. Rather, we endeavour to avoid it or any semblance of it. It is too incalculable a factor for the physician who desires to realise, as far as may be, what he is doing. That does not mean that he dare shut his eyes to its existence, but he can at least avoid anything that appears to encourage it, unless it is intended deliberately to use its therapeutic power.

With these comments the way is now clear for a statement of the actual results obtained. We have classified them as Excellent, Good, Moderate and Negative, the last being those of complete failure. Let the last be considered first. They are not concerned with any special variety of disease. For every case that has failed we can show numbers of apparently similar cases that have succeeded. It is not even always the cases most obviously of long standing and severity that do not respond. Frequently cases that seem to offer little ground for hope do well and others of apparently less severe a type prove disappointing. Here, for instance, is a case of chronic headache.

Miss X had suffered all her life from severe headaches occurring on an average twice a month. No treatment had helped her to any marked extent. An organism was found and she received two doses (2 millions and 4 millions respectively) with an interval of seven weeks between them. After each dose there was a distinct aggravation of symptoms lasting two weeks,—then a return to the previous condition, but not improvement. Yet chronic headache as will be presently seen is one of the disorders wherein we have scored most brilliant successes. Similarly we have seldom failed to do something, though often slowly, for chronic arthritis, but we have to record several failures ; the same is true of skin diseases though there is a special difficulty with these disorders. Frequently the sufferers are not ill " in themselves " (rather as though the skin trouble hindered the development of deeper symptoms), but anxious to be rid of a disfigurement. As the

first effect of a dose is often to increase this
and as this aggravation is often rather
prolonged, it is only natural that the patient
becomes restive and seeks relief elsewhere.
We have cases that have finally done very
well indeed, but these were of the more
patient kind of citizen and willing to wait.
It is most desirable to follow the histories
of chronic skin lesions over long periods
of years, to determine whether or no the
sufferers are relatively free of other chronic
diseases and whether, when their skin
troubles are markedly relieved by external
applications there is any tendency for other
symptoms (headache, dyspepsia, lassitude,
joint pains and so forth) to appear. The
skin is held by Professor Much and his
followers to be the organ *par excellence* for
the development of anti-bodies. Are manifestations of skin disease possibly roundabout
attempts to establish an effective resistance
against deep bacterial infection ? If it were
so, it would be easy to understand why a

vaccine dose should cause a temporary worsening, because the system being already in the way of using the skin defensively proceeds readily to use it a little more for this purpose.

Epilepsy again is a disease wherein we have obtained successes—yet here is a case of failure. Miss Y, 22 years old, who had suffered from epileptic attacks for years, increasing in frequency latterly in spite of various forms of treatment, came under observation. In this disease we generally find a Proteus type of organism, but in this lady the bacteria were more of the Gærtner type. The results of using a vaccine however were entirely negative. There was no marked aggravation of symptoms and no improvement. Several doses were given at intervals before treatment was abandoned.

It is impossible not to endeavour to discover the causes of failure. First and foremost, naturally, we have to face the fact that a vaccine is designed to encourage a response for which the body already possesses (presumably) the necessary mechanism. But there must occasionally be cases wherein there is no power of response existing and such cases are clearly beyond the range of the vaccine. More often probably the power is there but cannot be used because of some hindering influence. Just as we believe that non-lactose-fermenting organisms are often the influence that hinders the action of a vaccine made from a nasal or pelvic focus, so possibly sometimes there ie a secondary infection able to hinder the work of an intestinal vaccine. At any rate all failures should be carefully investigated from this point of view. Further, although in many cases the vaccine will do much without strict dieting, it is always worth while with a failure to put the patient on a strict diet (See Appendix A) and then, after an interval try the vaccine again. Too large a dosage and too frequent repetition are causes of many disappointing results but they will be better considered in relation to the class of moderate success. If nevertheless one or two of the usual doses produce no favourable result and no reaction, it is worth while (especially after a period of dieting) to try the effect of a much larger initial dose. It is quite possible that some drugs may be found capable of preparing the system better to receive the vaccine stimulus. Sulphur particularly and Iodine are worthy of consideration in this respect.

Finally (and this applies also to the class of Moderate Success) there are cases which will respond to a polyvalent vaccine and not to an autogenous. The phenomenon suggests that the autogenous vaccine may sometimes be too nearly identical with the pre-existing chronic invader to stimulate the system and the slightly more removed polyvalent vaccine more suitable. At any rate, the phenomenon appears now and then and it is worth while to remember its existence and try a polyvalent vaccine if an autogenous fails or disappoints. Of the 467 cases which are here under consideration, we have to class 23 as failures, a percentage of 4.9.

We can now take the next class, those wherein there has been a definite and favourable response to treatment, but wherein the improvement has stopped short of a cure or even of very notable permanent relief so that the final results can only be classed as Moderate. This is in many ways a most disappointing class. Naturally a rheumatoid arthritis with marked bony changes is beyond cure and any improvement here is a gain, but there are other cases wherein there has been enough improvement to rouse great hopes and then for no obvious reason a failure to progress any further.

Much that has been said concerning the total failures has an application also for this class of moderate success. But stress must be laid on one factor already alluded to which particularly concerns these cases. It is the factor of dosage too large or of repeti-

tion too frequent. The latter is the more
insidious enemy. There is no harm in
beginning with a very small dose. We
suggest 2 millions but even less might be given
if desired. For if there is no response at all
then after an interval of not less than three
to four weeks (sometimes even less) a larger
quantity can be injected. But too frequent
repetition may ruin the most promising
beginnings. The ideal is to give a dose,
obtain its full effect and allow the effect to
begin to pass off. In other words, if there
is a favourable response, do not repeat until
it is certain that the improvement has come
to an end. Whether the waiting stage has
to be six weeks or six months, there should
be no wavering in obedience to this rule.
But physicians and patients are human and
therefore impatient and the cure of chronic
disease is, at the best, apt to be slow. The
abiding terror of the physician is to incur
even a suspicion of keeping a patient under
treatment for his own gain longer than is

necessary. This fear is one of the burdens laid on the profession by a social organisation which compels us to sell health for money in order to live and it is a very real burden. It is in consequence of this that it is so difficult to resist the hope that a process of recovery can be hastened " and striving to better oft we mar what's well." For instance Mr. Z had suffered for the greater part of his life, over thirty years, from attacks of depression during which all power of mental concentration was so diminished that he could only keep at work with great difficulty, while any zest for life not unnaturally disappeared. After a period of weeks or months (seldom less than four to five weeks) the cloud would lift quite suddenly and there would be a period of complete (apparent) health. On an average every year would bring at least two of these attacks of depression and no treatment (though many were tried) availed to give any real relief. There would be bad days and days not so bad, but in spite of all efforts patience until the attack passed off was the principal resource. When he came under treatment an organism was readily found and the first dose was given during one of the periods of depression. The effect was almost immediate. The patient within 24 hours was completely relieved. To find a remedy capable of bringing his misery to an end was a new experience and it was not unnatural that he should decide that he would have recourse to it without delay in the next emergency. But the very confidence that a remedy had been found tempted him to use it on slight provocation, without any delay to discover whether the first symptoms of renewed depression really pointed to a severe return of his trouble or no. Consequently he clamoured for doses which were in our judgment too frequent, always insisting that without them he would be left in unbearable and unjustifiable misery. It was very difficult to assess the real immi-

nence of an attack and almost impossible
to refuse the remedy without incurring the
self-reproach of which we spoke above.
For a time we tried to avoid danger by
giving minimal doses. We gave *placebos*
now and then but they were without effect,
countering the explanation that suggestion
alone accounted for the improvement. For
a time the doses were effective, but before
long they lost all power and ultimately the
old condition was re-established and the
vaccine treatment remained only a disappointing memory. Actually, with the
best intentions we had " immunized " him
against his vaccine and his system would
no longer respond. He has long ceased
vaccine treatment and it is difficult to say
whether he has received any permanent
gain from it. Possibly had he been willing
to wait for some months on a strict diet
he might have recovered some power of
response and possibly a polyvalent vaccine
might have been of value, but with such

knowledge as we then possessed we were not confident in urging this course nor was the patient in his natural disappointment very inclined to take our advice. This therefore is a case where it is difficult to resist the judgement that there was some favourable effect produced but the net result was disappointing. Others in this class, while unsatisfactory, are rather better than this example. For instance, Mr. F had suffered from Psoriasis for seventeen years (body and head). He had 5 doses from September 1918 to May 1919. There was steady improvement until the area affected was diminished by fifty per cent., but thereafter further treatment has failed to produce any effective result.

In this class we have to place 68 cases out of the 467 or 14.5 per cent. In all probability further experience and the knowledge it brings will enable us to improve upon these figures, but even now less than twenty per cent. of all our cases fall into these two classes of complete failure and slight or temporary improvement.

We can now turn to the more encouraging side of our results. The good cases we divide into two classes—the excellent and remarkable recoveries ; and the ones that make good but slower and less dramatic progress. In this last class, called " Good " cases, we include such instances as these that follow.

Mr. M, aged forty, had suffered for seven years from persistent Psoriasis of head and body. He received doses from July, 1922 to June, 1923—five in all. In October, 1922 the Psoriasis had virtually disappeared. In April, 1923, there was a slight return and he received his fourth dose then. After the fifth, in June 1923, no more treatment has been required and there has been (to date) no sign of the disease.

Mr. F, aged 48, suffered from Psoriasis of legs and arms for fifteen years. He received in all five doses from March 1922, to September 1923. Great improvement followed from the first three doses ; the last two were given for a slight return, cleared up the condition entirely and there has been no recurrence.

Mr. F. W, aged 17, had suffered from epileptic attacks for some years before coming under treatment. As many as six attacks in one week were recorded (of a severe type and) he also stammered very badly. There was no improvement rather the contrary on Bromides. He received eight doses between December, 1921 and October, 1923. He has had no attack since December 1923, his stammering is much less and no Bromide has been given for two years.

Mr. L was a chronic dyspeptic of six years standing, in whom colitis had been diagnosed. His symptoms were indigestion, abdominal pain and loss of appetite, some mucus and some blood in the stools. Four doses were given from May, 1919 to July 1920. All symptoms by then had disappeared and there has been no return of them up to the present date.

Mr. K had suffered for three years from great mental depression, accompanied by very severe pain in the back of the neck and shoulders. He received eight doses from February 1919 to April 1923. Since October 1920, he has been free of all symptoms, except that in June 1921 and April 1923 a slight return led to the administration of further doses. None have been required since the last date nearly two years ago.

Mr. K. S had suffered from recurrent attacks of Sciatica for years. When he came under treatment he had endured an acute attack for six weeks. He received five doses from February 1922 to June 1923. There has been no serious pain since April 1922, though slight symptoms were met by renewed doses January and June 1923. Since then no pain has been felt.

Mrs. H, aged 66, had suffered from

Rheumatoid Arthritis for 20 years. For three years before coming under treatment, she had been unable to walk. Typical deformities were present in hands, knees and feet. Great depression and pain were present. Six doses were given in 1921, three in 1922, two in 1923 and one in 1924. She began to improve at once and has steadily progressed. No severe pain has been felt since June 1921. At present the deformity is about a quarter of the original extent. She can use her hands and arms and walk half a mile ; she has no depression and no pain.

Mrs. P, aged 33, had had headaches most of her life and for five years, before coming under treatment, a severe attack once a week necessitating rest in bed for 24 hours. She has had six doses from September 1923 to December 1924. The last severe headache was in May, 1924 and her general health has improved very greatly.

The above are fair samples of the kind

of case which we class as a good result and in this division we place 309 cases, being 66.1 per cent. The remainder of our cases, 67 in number or 14.3 per cent., can only be described as remarkable and brilliant successes. It is impossible to prophesy at present which cases will respond as rapidly and completely as these have done, but the phenomenon is very gratifying for patient and physician and further knowledge may enable us to foresee its possibility and even to encourage its appearance. We append a few instances to give an idea of the kind of case which we class in this division.

Mr. D. working in India, had suffered, from mild Dysenteric Colitis for some years. In the summer of 1923 Sugar appeared in the urine to the extent of 4 per cent. Wasting and thirst were prominent symptoms and in 1924 the patient was given a year's leave to try the effect of treatment in England. He received vaccine doses in June, July and September, 1924. Improvement was rapid from the first, he gained in weight, lost his thirst and as at the end of September all trace of Sugar had disappeared and he was in excellent health, he returned to India. Up to the last report (January, 1925) he has remained perfectly well and there is no trace of Glycosuria.

Mrs. W, for three years had suffered from Glycosuria up to 4 per cent. with neuritis and a blood pressure of 225 c.m.m. She received a dose on January 19th 1924 and on February 7th the B.P. was 168 and no sugar could be detected. She is perfectly well to date, March 1925.

Mr. B, aged 44, developed epileptic attacks sixteen months before coming under vaccine treatment. In spite of Bromides, etc., the attacks became more severe and more frequent (two a week finally) and he was pensioned off by his firm as incurable. All Bromide was stopped and he received his first two doses of vaccine on November

10th 1918 and January 6th 1919. The severe attacks ceased after the first dose, though attacks of the *petit mal* type occurred occasionally. In February 1919 he resumed work and with no holiday continued without missing a day for 18 months. The *petit mal* attacks disappeared in February 1919 until June, 1920. Then on his reporting a mild return (*petit mal*) a third dose was given. From that time until he was last seen, June 1924, there has been no attack of any kind and he has enjoyed perfect general health.

Mr. T, aged 52, reported " not one day of health since 1906 " and when seen was in a state of profound mental depression, afraid to cross the road, afraid of noise, intensely irritable and suffering from persistent insomnia. The first dose of vaccine was given on May 4th 1920 with an immediate disappearance of all symptoms. A slight return of depression and fear led to the giving of the second dose on June 24th,

1920, seven weeks later. The result was all that could be desired. At the end of June (within a week) the patient went to Holland by aeroplane (an inconceivable feat for him in his earlier condition) and has remained perfectly well since.

Mr. C. B suddenly discovered that he was losing the sight of his left eye. Tobacco Amblyopia was diagnosed and treated for six months ; at the end of that time the left eye was no better, the right eye was affected so that he could not read headlines in a newspaper and found it dangerous to cross a road. Early fundus changes were reported. On February 10th 1920 the first dose of vaccine was given. Improvement set in at once. Soon large print was read with ease. On June 1st the second dose was given and within three days he could read small print and has had no return of any eye trouble up to the present time.

Miss J for nine months before vaccine treatment had suffered from very severe pain at the back of the neck extending down the left arm. Pain prevented sleep. Neuritis had been diagnosed. The first and only dose was given on October 14th 1924. Pain disappeared in twenty-four hours and has not returned up to the present time, March 1925.

Mr. W, 40 years old, reported attacks of Sciatica in the right leg with violent cramp, for the last twenty years. He had had to remain in bed for as much as two weeks at a time and for the last two years the intervals between attacks were lessening and a few weeks respite was as much as he enjoyed. He received two doses on June 16th 1924 and August 20th 1924. The pain disappeared at once and has not returned (March, 1925) a longer interval of freedom than he has known for twenty years.

Mr. F, came for treatment February 1923, with a history of recurrent colitis since 1915, constant diarrhœa and nausea with more violent attacks about once a month. On February 13th 1923, he received his first and only dose, improved at once and has been entirely well ever since.

Mr. D, aged 54, came with early Rheumatoid Arthritis of finger and toe joints, wrists, elbows, hips and worst of all, knees. He reported the condition as getting steadily worse and walking was increasingly painful and difficult. He was very depressed mentally. The first dose was given on April 13th 1919. Rapid improvement ensued. Further doses were given on June 7th and August 3rd 1919 and by this time the condition of all the joints had returned to normal health. A slight return of pain led to the administration of another dose in June 1924, and no further treatment has been required.

Mrs. B, aged 68, described chronic headaches, affecting her for forty years. For the first ten years they occurred about twice a month ; for the next ten years once a week and for the last twenty years she had spent as a rule three days in bed in each week on account of them. The patient was wasted and ill and described her life as " unbearable." On December 7th 1920 she received her first dose and thereafter had no bad headache for a year and gained 16 pounds in weight. A second dose was given on December 10th 1921, and there has been no headache of any importance since then.

These cases are enough to show the character of our class marked excellent, and we repeat that they number 67 or 14.3 per cent. Together with the class of thoroughly good results they amount virtually to 80 per cent. of the whole and we contend that that is too high a proportion (considering the serious chronic conditions which make up our series), to allow the vaccines to be disregarded as agents of cure. At least the figures make difficult the use of such words as suggestion or coincidence, or the other excuses which are apt to be

murmured by those disinclined to undertake
the experiments by which alone a true
judgement can be obtained.

Finally, there must be some statement
as to the varieties of chronic disease treated.
They include every kind of chronic arthritis, rheumatic, rheumatoid and gouty,
cases of Psoriasis and chronic Eczema,
colitis and chronic dyspepsia. There are
cases of chronic illness the sequels of
Tubercular affections though we are
careful of possible aggravations whenever
there is reason to think that there is any
active focus of disease. Among nervous
diseases, epilepsy accounts for some cases
and in the field of neurasthenia we have
scored heavily on many occasions. Instances of chronic headaches have been
given and there are many of them and
even cases bordering on mental disease
(especially melancholia) have frequently responded well. The cases of malignant
disease are dealt with in the chapter that

follows and there are stray instances of a
large number of other chronic conditions
which encourage the hope that whenever
in a chronic disease an intestinal organism is
found (and that is virtually always if due
search is made), it is worth while to try a
vaccine made from it, as it may well prove
to be at least one of the decisive factors in
bringing about recovery or marked improvement. We are well aware that the
good cases may sound almost too good to
be true—yet we have observed nearly all
of them over long periods of time and we
have made no attempt in any way to select
the series of five hundred. It is at first
sight extraordinary that such swift and
dramatic improvement should, even now
and then, ensue in diseases that have lasted
for months and years. But the records
show that it can happen and that in 80 per
cent. of all cases striking benefit is obtained.
Perhaps we should rather conclude that if
a few, well spaced, doses of vaccine can

achieve so much, so often, the capacity of the human body to develop resistance to these chronic enemies is not only generally present, but readily stimulated. That is a very hopeful thought : for by judicious treatment in the early stages these disorders should be prevented from ever becoming chronic and a careful prophylaxis may in time reduce the incidence of these most troublesome ills to a fraction of their present number and very likely prolong life in perfect health to a length that to-day sounds all but incredible.

CHAPTER V.

IT was inevitable that the problem of
Cancer should come to be considered
as soon as results began to be obtained
in the cure and relief of other chronic
diseases. This book would be incomplete
without a discussion of the possible relation
of *Cancer* to *Intestinal Infections* and some
account of the results which we have obtained in this disease by the use of vaccines.

It may be fairly said of cancer, in the
present state of knowledge, that it is an
ultimate condition, a final result to which
a number of factors have contributed. It
is as yet impossible to speak dogmatically
as to the relative weight to be attached to
any one of these factors. But although the
recent attempts to select (*e.g.*) meat-eating,
or improper diet in general, as the main

cause of Cancer can hardly be said to be proved, enough evidence has been accumulated to make it highly probable that poisoning from the alimentary canal is a factor of importance.

It has been made sufficiently clear by now that in our opinion diet is important in relation to intestinal toxæmia, in proportion as it encourages or discourages the growth of intestinal organisms of the non-lactose-fermenting groups. In this respect merely to be a vegetarian is not a complete safeguard. The factor of cooking in diet is of the utmost importance and it would be possible to be a vegetarian of the strictest sect and yet be doing little or nothing to inhibit bacterial intestinal growth.

Further, once these infections are established, it is not according to our experience that diet *alone* will eradicate them. It is of the greatest service as an addition to vaccines, but seldom if ever more than palliative alone. Again it may be said of potassium starvation that very likely it plays a part, but a subsidiary part. Forced thus, as we have been, to regard diet alone as an incomplete treatment for the disease of Cancer, we investigated the bacteriology of the fæces of the cancerous. Non-lactose-fermenting organisms are easily found in all cases and we proceeded to test the effects of vaccines made from them.

Practically all the cases dealt with have been of the inoperable type and almost all of inoperable recurrences, in a very advanced condition and yet more than sixty per cent. of these have shown relief of symptoms and general and local improvement to a definite degree.

Those cases which have come to us to be treated without an operation have been refused, as we feel that complete removal, when possible, still offers the best chance of cure. But vaccine treatment has been given after removal of the growth in the hope that it might prove effective as prophylactic against recurrence. There is reason to believe that this is a hopeful procedure, for in some cases, where the prognosis was decidedly bad owing to imperfect removal of the tumour, health has been maintained for considerable periods and in a few cases suspicious nodules left after the operation have disappeared.

If, as we can show, intestinal cleansing can in a definite percentage of hopeless cases effect some relief and in certain other cases diminution of growth, how much more effective should this be in the earliest stages of the disease, or still more as a preventive of its occurrence ?

When it has been possible, a strict diet has been combined with the administration of the vaccines, but for economic reasons in institutional work this cannot always be done, and we have found that although diet undoubtedly is of importance, yet definite and striking results may be obtained with vaccination alone.

The interval of dosing is the same as for chronic disease generally ; doses are only repeated when indicated by the condition of the patient. In the majority of cases pain, hæmorrhage or local symptoms have been the guide for repetition, but in cases where there is little or no local trouble, the general condition of the patient is taken into account.

In connection with malignant disease (as sometimes occurs in other chronic disorders), a polyvalent vaccine of the type of organism found in the patient is more effective than an autogenous preparation. This can only be discovered by dealing with each case individually and though it is difficult to assign any reason for the fact, it is surprising how even when the fæces may show an almost pure culture of an abnormal bacillus, the polyvalent vaccine is more effective than the autogenous.

The reaction which occurs in cases of malignant disease after an inoculation not only affects the general health, increasing malaise, weakness etc., for a few hours or days, but also causes an increase of those symptoms directly attributable to the new growth itself. A corresponding ameliora-ation follows and in many cases this is most marked, especially as regards pain. It is difficult to conceive why the effect of the vaccine is often most marked upon the pain which so frequently accompanies Cancer.* But it is to the relief of that symptom that we look most confidently. Morphia can often be all but dispensed with, when vaccine treatment is employed and even when the cases slowly sink and die, the relief to the last months or weeks of suffering is in itself by no means to be despised.

As has already been stated, it is only with hopeless, inoperable cases that we have

*It is possible that the pain of malignant disease is actually dependent upon the extension of it. As a new area is invaded, pain is one of the reactions to the invasion. Since we are confident that vaccines at least check the rate of new growth, it may be in this way that they relieve suffering in so marked a manner.

been dealing. So far no cure has been recorded, but the great majority are markedly relieved from symptoms, improve in general health and life is prolonged probably by months. The main benefit so far lies in that the patient has a much more comfortable time. The end, when it comes, is generally sudden, following a relapse, often alas ! when they have begun to feel that there is even some hope of being cured.

If this can be done in hopeless cases, how much more hopeful should be the outlook if vaccine treatment is begun early ? It is, perhaps, not too optimistic to look forward to the day when we shall dare to take an early case even out of the hands of the surgeon.

We have had cases where a tumour has been reduced to half its size, others where pain ceases a few hours after inoculation, others where œdema has disappeared in an extraordinary way, and apart from these striking results we have had a large number of cases where there has been some definite, though not so brilliant, benefit. It must always be remembered that we have so far treated none but hopeless and terminal cases. If other investigators can confirm our results, it will be justifiable to make a vaccine treatment the ordinary sequel to operation and even perhaps now and then to give it a chance before operation. When it works it works quickly so that there need be no long delay. In the realm of pure prophylaxis obviously much remains to be done before any opinion can be even hinted at. Only if (and when) these intestinal infections come to be largely recognised as of importance and suitably treated, then if they have anything serious to contribute towards the causation of Cancer, there should be a sensible diminution in the amount of malignant disease. That is all that can be said now and only the work of future years can give the final answer to the problem.

We append the results of treatment in a

series of 33 cases of malignant disease. It is only during the last few years that we have attempted to influence Cancer and we cannot include any case which has not been under observation for a period of six months at least. Nevertheless the results obtained are of interest. There has been no selection of cases ; they have been taken as they came. Again we must insist that every one of them was regarded, when treatment was begun, as hopeless, with only a brief period of life to be anticipated. All were inoperable, many of them recurrences after operation.

As before we make four classes ; those that have progressed very well indeed, those that have made substantial improvement, those showing some, but not marked gain and those that have not responded at all. We will now give in brief detail an example of each class in order to establish the standards which govern each division. First, this is the kind of result which we class as very good.

Mr. X. aged 48, had been treated for six months as a case of nervous dyspepsia, but on examination in October, 1924, a large growth over the gall bladder region and involving the liver was readily discovered. Oedema was marked in both legs, dysphagia present to such an extent that only fluids could be swallowed, there was cough with blood-stained sputum and dull patches in both lungs, extreme depression and great loss of weight—two stone in six months. A cautious prognosis would have given him about two months to live. To-day, March 1925, the growth in the liver is definitely though slightly diminished and every other disease symptom has completely disappeared. The cough has ceased, the dysphagia has vanished and there is no trace of œdema. The patient refuses to consider himself an invalid and has gained fifteen pounds in weight. He has had two doses, October 1924 and January 1925, and the greater part of the troublesome symptoms disappeared within ten days of the first dose. The indication for the January dose was a return of the mental depression.

Of our cases treated twelve per cent. are of this class.

In the second class we place cases of the following type :

Mrs. C. aged 34, right breast removed twelve months earlier for advanced carcinoma. On examination the liver was found enlarged and nodular, fluid present in both pleural cavities, consolidated patches above the fluid, sternum bulging and extensive growth in the walls of the chest. Pain was severe, vomiting frequent, respirations hurried (30) and pulse 120. This was on March 15th 1922, when the first dose was given. Twenty-four hours afterwards vomiting was relieved, respirations had dropped to 22 and pulse to 90. Pain was very much less. Steady improvement ensued till April 30th, when the patient was able to be up and about and do a little gardening which she loved. The second dose on April 30th was given because the condition had remained stationary for two weeks. Another spurt of benefit followed and until September the patient lived virtually a normal life. The fluid had long since disappeared from the chest, although the growth had only slightly diminished. But there was no pain or other untoward symptom. In September 1922, the third dose was given for some return of pain. Improvement again followed until December 16th, when bronchitis developed, the result of a " cold," and the patient died suddenly on December 26th. Here, as in so many of these advanced cases, life has only been made much pleasanter and more prolonged, but in so striking a manner that it is impossible not to credit the vaccine with a marked effect. It is no small matter for patient and friends when a state of misery is swiftly changed to one of peace and relative ease. To all intents and purposes this lady led her normal life for the last six or seven months of her existence.

Of such cases we number fifty per cent., so that with the foregoing class we can say that sixty-two per cent. of the total have responded well.

In the third class we have to place twenty-eight per cent. of our cases and they conform to the following type :

Mr. W. S. was a case of inoperable recurrence of carcinoma of the tongue, with a tumour the size of a walnut in the floor of the mouth and marked sub-maxillary glands on both sides. Pain was severe, necessitating sedatives. Slight hæmorrhage from the growth occurred every day. The first dose was given on November 7th 1923. After 24 hours all pain and hæmorrhage ceased. The growth diminished slightly in size in the following weeks. On December 5th a second dose was given as the condition remained stationary. There was little or no change though pain and hæmorrhage remained absent. On January 29th, 1924, as there was slight return of pain, a third dose was given and the pain ceased again. The growth now began slowly to increase in size and on March 1st the patient died quite suddenly, apparently of heart failure. No sedatives were given from November 8th to the time of death.

There remain ten per cent. of cases wherein vaccines have been of no avail and no improvement whatever has followed their use.

We need not here repeat the arguments already used that if these results can be obtained in such desperate and final cases the prospects of earlier treatment should be brighter. Much work obviously remains to be done, for as yet we cannot be sure that with vaccines for chronic intestinal infections we are dealing with more than one of the factors whose combined influence results in malignant disease. But at least we claim that these results are sufficient to suggest the importance of this toxæmic factor and the advisability of endeavouring to combat it.

.

CHAPTER VI.

THE work of the Medical Profession is two-fold : To prevent diseases in the community and to cure it in individual cases. The last hundred years have seen great successes achieved in the prevention of disease, but as regards cure of existing disorders, while there have been many striking individual results, there is a long road yet to travel before the ideal of the profession is fully attained.

Since the final object of all treatment in disease is cure or at least relief, the final test of any method is the result of it upon the patient. No amount of laboratory evidence or theoretical argument will suffice to overcome clinical failure. Nevertheless the physician who depends almost entirely (as we do) upon clinical results in support of his theories must be prepared to face a certain amount of doubt. For the capacity of cases to recover independently of any treatment, can never, in the present state of our knowledge, be accurately estimated and the fact that cure follows a certain procedure never establishes more than a presumption that the treatment was efficacious. Single cases offer no proof. The history of medicine is strewn thick with vaunted treatments which have failed to establish their claims and there is no patent medicine-vendor or advertised miracle worker, no manipulator, no dietician or exercise professor who cannot show among his results genuine recoveries from genuine diseases. To apportion rightly the claims to success of the multifarious treatments of to-day demands more searching analysis and more patient investigation, than any individual practitioner can give. Therefore, he is apt to be swayed in his judgement by his initial experiences. If they show success he will use the treatment, for patients demand cures and the practitioner must endeavour to supply them.

We are only too well aware therefore that our hypothesis concerning the nature of chronic disease can be no more than a hypothesis until it has received a very careful and widespread testing. Indeed it is precisely in order that it may receive such a testing that this book has been written. But vaccine therapy in general appears well established and has justified itself to the judgement of the profession. Consequently in associating the constant presence of certain organisms with the symptoms of various chronic diseases and in using vaccines of them for the relief of these maladies, it is possible to appeal to the general faith in vaccine treatment as a reason for experiment in these further instances. It may also be urged that if (as some hold) these organisms are non-pathogenic, then a vaccine made from them will at least be unlikely to do any harm and the experiment can be undertaken without fear. True, it will mean the injection of foreign protein, but on the other hand we suggest, indeed we urge, such small and infrequent doses that any conceivable risk is minimal.

Further, in appealing to clinical results, we lay stress on the frequency of favourable response. If an organism of this type is discovered and a vaccine administered, we confidently expect *some* favourable result in 90 per cent. of all cases. Naturally complete cure is slow (though we expect some improvement soon) and there are many cases which achieve a considerable advance, but do not reach the condition of entire recovery. But the cases which are entirely refractory are a small minority and if our results can be confirmed by other investigators, it will become increasingly difficult to regard them as accidental and fallacious.

It is worth while to try to analyse the less favourable results as more is often to be learnt from failure than from success. The first and obvious difficulty is that of chronicity. So many cases do not attempt treatment until years of poisoning have wrought tissue changes which may well be irremediable and advancing life in itself means a lessening power of response to stimuli. If treatment could be early (or even prophylactic), infinitely better results should be obtainable and old age itself might turn out to be largely a toxæmia, to be deferred and mitigated by appropriate treatment.

A second factor which may cause relative failure is of deep interest. We have already suggested that one of the earlier effects of these chronic toxæmias with which we are concerned is lowering of resistance to other organisms. Consequently a case of chronic disease frequently shows not only an intestinal organism, but also some other local infection, streptococcal, pneumococcal or whatever. Our belief is that efficient protec ion against the deep infection from the first (accompanied possibly by certain care in diet) would have prevented the secondary infection and in some cases the result of a vaccine directed against the primary invader enables the system to deal also with the latter without more ado. But these cases are a minority. Once a secondary invader is established, usually it needs to be dealt with also by means of its own appropriate vaccine. The two vaccines can be administered together.

Care in the due consideration of these two factors will enhance the physician's success and incidentally and by degrees knowledge may be gained as to which secondary infections are the most serious and hindering. Finally, in any refractory case, it is well worth while to try a rigid dieting (fruit, vegetables, nuts and dairy produce) for some weeks and then give the vaccine another chance. The relative cleansing of the bowel often makes just the necessary difference for enabling success to be attained.

Before considering briefly the place of
accessory treatments, a word may be said
to meet one obvious objection to our
hypothesis. It may well be urged : " You
suggest that faulty diet predisposes to these
chronic infections and draw a direful picture
of the combined results of diet and disease,
but the diet has been that of man (more or
less) for centuries, and yet in spite of it he
has multiplied and made our civilization.
Is there not some disproportion between
your picture of all but universal disease and
man's actual achievement ? " The objection requires some answer. In the first
place, it may well be replied that all that
man has achieved has been done in spite of,
not in absence of, a great deal of disease.
There is no record in history of a civilized
race immune from disease and it is notorious
that many of the greatest names on the roll
of mankind are those of men suffering from
disease, often dying young. There is no
proportional relation between health and

mental achievement, although hard, muscular work requires physical "fitness." There is a fascinating bye-path to explore in the problem whether disease may not sometimes be an actual temporary stimulus to intellectual achievement. It seems to be a universal rule that any agent which damages or destroys in a relatively large dose, stimulates life activity in a relatively small one. The first effects, therefore, of the chronic toxæmia which we postulate might be to encourage brain activity while the dosage of poison is yet small. Naturally it is not suggested that it will turn a poor brain into a good one, but it may for a time encourage the activity of both and when the brain is good, important work may result. We have known at least one case wherein a brain worker found his inventive faculties considerably lessened *pari passu* with response otherwise favourable to vaccine treatment. In the long last of course real health conduces to the best work of all kinds.

No one would deliberately seek ill-health as a stimulus, since the dosage of it is uncontrollable.

Returning to the main theme, it must also be said that during the first thirty or forty years of life, there is an elasticity, a reserve of power which keeps in the background the symptoms of chronic disease and for a time even the infected may appear to be models of physical and mental health. Therefore, the achievements of the race are not in themselves any disproof that our ancestors, even as we, were not subject to these toxæmias. Nature is in any case " careless of the single life." These diseases do not threaten life urgently and provided that a due proportion of the race survives to rear offspring, the disabilities of the individual are not much regarded by whatever powers rule our destinies.

Further, we have over and over again laid stress on the question of diet and are not yet done with it. Our ancestors in many ways had a fresher and simpler fare (with plenty of exceptions for special classes at special times), and often a larger proportion of uncooked or lightly cooked food. The ordinary Athenian citizen's diet of grain, olives, figs, cheese was plain living, but may well have helped the high thinking of his marvellous city : and there are plenty of races and civilizations whose diet it would be instructive to compare with their achievements. In our own day, there has been an enormous increase in the consumption of preserved foods (tinned, frozen or with added chemicals) and, for many classes, a lessening in the consumption of uncooked food. Much attention is being drawn to these food factors and their social importance to the community. We are not prepared to dogmatize against any but the use of chemicals in food (already condemned in the main by most expert opinions), and our views as to diet in general will presently either state or imply our attitude concerning these disputed matters.

We contend, therefore, that the human race may have suffered from these diseases, as Monsieur Jourdain spoke prose, without knowing it. It remains to consider what other treatment besides vaccines is available or desirable. Let a word be said first as to B. Coli infections. After years of testing we have come to believe that in the bowel B. Coli comes very near to being what our non-lactose-fermenting germs are believed by some to be, namely a non-pathogenic organism. Even if repeated examinations reveal no other bacillus we have seldom, if ever, seen vaccines of it improve the cases ; and finally, if enough examinations are made or a provocative injection of a stock vaccine of non-lactose-fermenting germs be given, another organism will be detected and is virtually always a much more hopeful enemy to attack. When, however, B. Coli makes its way (as so often) into the urinary tract and kidney, bladder, or prostate is markedly affected, the case is somewhat different.

Coli vaccines here will do much to clear the tract. But the disorder is very likely to recur. We regard it as a secondary invasion and should still press the search for a bowel organism of a deeper acting type. If one is found, then we regard a mixed vaccine made from the deeper acting organism and the B. Coli together, as the correct (and generally successful) weapon.

Among the accessory measures, diet, as already indicated more than once, holds the first place. The possibility that methods of food preservation play a part in intestinal infection has already been mentioned and in the present state of knowledge little more of value can be said. It is a question for future investigation. Setting it aside, we have no doubt that the more diet conforms to the type made up of fresh fruit salads, nuts, (very important) cereals, (wholemeal bread and raw oatmeal particularly) and dairy produce, with little or no tea, coffee or spirits, the healthier is the bowel likely to be in regard to non-lactose-fermenting organisms, to say nothing of products of putrefaction. But to the ordinary citizen this will be very much a counsel of perfection (not to say of dismay) and it is only in special cases that it is likely to be followed. There is little hope that mankind (European and American at least) will ever conform to it.* Incidentally, it may be said that merely to become a " vegetarian " as commonly understood is not in itself a guarantee of a good diet. Vegetarians avoid certain dangers but do not always consume enough uncooked food. For it is more than likely that cooking is as much to blame as the ingredients of diet themselves.

*There is a story concerning a poem on the subject of Nebuchadnezzar sent in for the Newdigate prize. It contained the following lines relative to the monarch's madness and the consequent change in his diet :—

" He murmured as he chewed the unwonted food
'It may be wholesome, but it is not good ' "—

This aptly expresses the feeling of the ordinary, well-to-do patient when confronted with our dietetic suggestions in anything like rigour. The unqualified miracle-workers obtain obedience in matters such as these much more easily than the qualified physician, because by the nature of their position the public (half unconsciously) believes them to possess knowledge hidden from the profession and expect their recommendations to be odd and possibly unpleasant.

Nevertheless the race is not going to abandon the art of cooking and a way round the obstacle must be found.

This can be done. While we have every reason to believe that our remote ancestors developed the alimentary system which we inherit on uncooked food, yet cooking in some form has been practised for centuries and centuries. It has, we believe, brought in its train a greater liability to intestinal infections, but as these are slow and chronic they have not prevented the continuation of the race and when once he has generated his successors Nature has cared little for such ailments as merely make the individual uncomfortable. But judging from the response to vaccines, the mechanism of resistance to these infections exists ; if it has been evolved, the line of future progress will consist in so encouraging it that our bodies will pass from toleration of these organisms to active warfare against them, until a race shall develop capable of dealing with them while continuing to practise cookery and to eat a mixed diet.

In our experience diet alone however rigid will not eradicate these organisms if once they are established.* It will improve health and any obstinate case that proves refractory to vaccine treatment should invariably try the effect of rigid dieting for weeks. Thereafter vaccine therapy may, and probably will, prove more successful. But for the majority of cases this drastic dieting is unnecessary. Spirits should be abolished : twice cooked food condemned utterly : a proportion of uncooked food added to the dietary and raw fruit, salad, raw oatmeal and above all nuts ordered with insistence. This done, a vaccine will generally suffice. Fish, by the

*It is for this reason mainly that we hold that although poisoning by food derivatives may play a part in these chronic diseases, it cannot account for the whole of the phenomena. Rigid dieting will eliminate the food derivatives, but the patients (while improving) do not get well and the organisms remain until a vaccine is used. Then in many cases the germs disappear and the remaining symptoms with them. It is difficult to resist the belief that bacterial toxins, therefore, share in producing the disease.

way, seems a food rather better than meat and the latter should be curtailed, though here again there would be less objection to raw meat. There are certain sanatorium experiences that point to a considerable value for raw meat. But civilized people seldom find it palatable.* After diet, the therapeutic measures of exercise, massage, the varieties of radiation treatment, sunlight and electricity, have all in their different ways a real and often a great value. They appear to influence general metabolism, so that they encourage excretion of toxins and also oxidation of waste product poisons, and in some (perhaps all) cases influence endocrine balance. The beneficial effects of sunlight at any rate are now notorious. However, while all members of the community are the better for some of these agents and while the young may seem to be kept in perfect health by fresh air, sunshine and exercise, we have no reason to

*In any case nine out of ten of the well-to-do eat too much and have a quite unnecessary surplus of material to deal with. With the poor it is much more a question of a faulty and mistaken dietary.

believe that by themselves they can eradicate
chronic infections or prevent their implanta-
tion. They are accessory measures for
treatment of the utmost value but not enough
without the specific powers which are at
present most easily evoked by vaccines.

The value of courses of treatment at Spas
is undoubted, although it is common experience that the benefits obtained are often
only temporary and other visits are required.
At Spas there are not only available the
possible influences on general metabolism
already discussed (the regular life, baths
and massage, diet and exercise, sunlight
or other radiations), but in addition various
drugs are taken according to the locality
chosen. Of these some are purgative and
purgative drugs will be considered separately in a moment. The remainder may
be classed as " alteratives " a blessed word
which commits the user to very little. It
is worth while to consider their possibilities
briefly.

Sulphur is certainly a drug that, in spa treatment, is generally admitted to be beneficial. Professor Schulz of Greifswald, in his Inorganic Materia Medica, claims to have shown that it is a stimulant to general metabolism. Its action on the bowel is familiar and it is conceivable that it may influence local conditions and inhibit to some extent bacterial growth, not directly, but indirectly through its effects on the tissue. Iron and Arsenic are both excreted through the lower bowel in part and in process of excretion may modify the local conditions. Some of their " tonic " effects may be achieved thus. Drugs that influence organs like the liver may play a part, and drugs like Iodine which affect endocrine balance may thus influence general resistance to bacteria. These are the slightest (not to say vaguest) of suggestions, but they indicate problems whose solution awaits the pharmacologist. The profession has a store of drug experience which is largely empirical. In certain conditions certain remedies have seemed effective. It would be interesting to study the most favoured ones to discover any evidence in favour, first of a possible influence on the alimentary tract, which might check bacterial growth and second of a possible enhancing of resistance to infection.

So-called intestinal antiseptics must be considered next. They are prized by many physicians, but in our experience they do not sterilize the alimentary tract ; indeed it is all but inconceivable that they should. The organisms which they can deal with are the superficial ones, mostly already in process of being shed. The danger comes from the germs actually in the bowel lining, which are less easily reached. But an antiseptic is, *ipso facto*, a protoplasmic poison. The attempt to find poisons exclusively bacterio-tropic are not yet entirely successful and every "antiseptic" drug will have a greater or less effect on the cells with which it comes in contact. For good or evil it will affect their life activities. Further, the same agent which ends life activity in a relatively large dose stimulates it in one relatively small So that the user of an " antiseptic " may be influencing tissue cells when he conceives himself to be only killing bacteria. In this way, in some cases, an intestinal antiseptic may be followed by good results (as many believe) and yet leave the tract far from sterilized. Obviously such good results are not likely to be permanent. For our part we hold that if the anti-bacterial powers of the body can be encouraged, the outlook is more hopeful than when a direct attack is attempted on the bacteria. Cure, even relief, proceeds best, as it were, from within outwards.

The need for the future is actually to count the bacterial colonies, obtainable by plating material from the fæces, under various treatments. Then we shall know whether drugs or intestinal antiseptics influence them at all. We have tried the experiment for vaccines and have recorded the results in an earlier chapter. The use of a vaccine (*pari passu* with clinical improvement) is followed first by a great increase and then a gradual decrease in the colonies obtainable, till ultimately the organisms may disappear.

Conceiving, as we do, that the bowel is the source of the chronic toxæmia which causes much chronic disease, it would seem at first sight that all that was necessary was free purgation to ensure that as little opportunity as possible is given for toxic absorption. But the essential problem is not so easily solved. We have seen that even a rigid diet which, in many people, without any drugs will produce almost uncomfortably free purgation and an absence of the putrefactive type of substances, yet does not suffice in itself to eliminate the non-lactose-fermenting bacteria if once firmly implanted, nor entirely to cure the disease symptoms, although great improvement in them · may ensue. And no mere purgatives will do any better while, being all substances foreign to the body, they may affect it injuriously in course of time. Olive oil, Agar and its preparations are free from these latter risks and very valuable as accessory measures in the earlier stages of treatment. Earlier, because the constipation is itself a symptom of the toxæmia and will improve as the toxæmia is lessened. But obviously there must be a reasonable and regular relief from the bowel and the necessary measures to obtain it must be used.

The role of Surgery remains to be considered. To excise the Colon removes a large area from which toxic absorption is possible, even if it does not itself eradicate the chronic bowel infections. Consequently the favourable results claimed for it can readily be granted. But it is too drastic for any but the very severe sufferers, and vaccine treatment will often render it unnecessary even then.

We are not prepared to dogmatize as to the part played by the infections which we are considering in acute appendicitis and duodenal ulcer. We believe them to be a predisposing factor, but much more extended observation is required for any certainty. The acute emergencies remain surgical and must be in a surgeon's hands. But when the emergency is passed, bowel infection should be sought for and treated if found. A chronically inflamed appendix may be a source of irritation and of this, and of other bowel conditions with which the surgeon often has to deal, it may be said that vaccine treatment may sometimes prevent the conditions from ever arising, and sometimes come to be considered as a complement to operation. Each case must be judged on its merits.

The tale is now nearly told and we hope that enough has been said to ensure that

wide-spread testing of the vaccine treatment
of these chronic infections which alone can
bring certainty as to the part which they
play. Obviously, if once the fundamental
relation between them and many forms of
chronic disease can be established, there
are a number of most interesting further
problems clamouring for investigation. For
instance, we find the organisms to be of
great variety: will it be possible to asso-
ciate definite types with definite disease
pictures, e.g., one type for chronic arthritis,
one for psoriasis and so forth? Hitherto
the only comment we can make, even
tentatively, is that when the nervous system
is predominantly affected, e.g., in epilepsy,
the proteus type is frequently (not invariably) present. The fermentation reactions
are the only distinguishing features at the
moment. They are tedious and expensive to
investigate and the aid of many workers is
required. Clinically, the type of organism
seems to matter little : we have no reason to

believe that the body is refractory to a vaccine of any one.

But it cannot be too much emphasised that our ten years' experience compels us to be dogmatic about the mode of administration. Unless doses of vaccine are separated by long intervals of time (a minimum of six to eight weeks even when there is no apparent reaction at all and, if there is any improvement, then an interval that lasts as long as the improvement continues), very little, if any, success will be attained.

The process of resistance to these organisms is a delicate plant and over-much or over-rapid stimulation hinders or destroys it. The physician can do much harm by repeating his doses too soon : he can hardly do anything but good by delaying between doses.

But even in this counsel, although it may sound unusual, there is nothing really new. That the purpose of vaccine therapy is to encourage body resistance and so deal (indirectly) with disease is fully understood and there is no new principle involved in conceiving that the time may vary during which the response to a stimulus may last. This was and is the meaning of vaccination based on the opsonic index, namely to repeat the dose when needed and not before. If the length of time for which we ask seems incredible, it must be remembered how chronic are the diseases, how small the natural unaided tendency to develop resistance to them.

In any case the matter is one for experiment and it is to experiment that we confidently appeal ; "Esperienza, ch' esser suol' fonte ai rivi di vostr' arti." Our own experiments have extended over ten years and we are naturally influenced by their results. But any physician who cares can acquire enough experience of his own to justify an opinion. When, and only when, testing has been long enough and widespread enough shall we be able to say not

" We believe " but " We know." It is in the confident hope that faith will become knowledge that we lay this record of experiment and its associated argument before the Profession as a hypothesis concerning the nature and best treatment of many chronic diseases. We hope that we have not marred by arrogance or over-statement a case whose importance concerns the whole world.

APPENDIX A.

IT is convenient to tabulate the dietary to which we refer frequently in the foregoing chapters as an accessory measure which may definitely enhance the effect of a vaccine and may sometimes make the difference between its success or failure.

It is by no means always necessary to insist on it and as to many people their food is one of their principal joys, it is often difficult to get them to adhere even to a modified diet. We give the strict form of it and modifications and relaxations can readily be permitted when cases are doing well. The items of vital importance are the uncooked nuts and cereals.

It is perhaps hardly necessary to add that certain diseases (*e.g.* diabetes) will need the well-known modifications of diet to suit them.

Breakfast.

Porridge with milk or cream. (Sugar, if desired).

Eggs lightly poached or boiled.

Wholemeal bread.

Toast.

Jams and Marmalade.

Fresh Fruit (Grape fruit particularly).

Nuts.

Orangeade or Lemonade.

Weak Tea.

Coffee.

Honey.

Luncheon.

Hors d'œuvres (Sardines, Vegetable Salads, etc.).

Vegetable Soups.

Oysters.

Egg Dishes.

Any vegetable, cooked or raw, Salad or dessert.

Fruit salads.

Milk Puddings.

Wholemeal bread or toast.

Fish, if necessary.

Cheese.

Afternoon Tea may be allowed provided no great amount of solid is taken and only weak tea.

Dinner. The same kind of food as luncheon.

The day's diet should contain at least two oranges, one lemon, nuts, other fresh fruit and oatmeal uncooked. This may be mixed with porridge or taken with cream or fruit juice or sprinkled on puddings.

In cases of Malignant Disease, we prefer that no meat should be taken.

Wearers of dental plates find nuts tiresome to masticate. But they can, of course, be grated or pounded beforehand, and there are various forms of crushed nuts on the market which are suitable.

APPENDIX B.

METHOD OF PREPARING VACCINES FROM THE
GRAM-NEGATIVE NON-LACTOSE-FERMENTING
BACILLI.

FORTUNATELY the abnormal organisms which we are anxious to obtain, generally survive for some time in the specimen after collection, and if present can usually be cultured after 48 hours even if the specimen has been kept in the cold, so that there is no urgent necessity to plate within a few hours of the stool being passed, though it is probably wise not to leave it longer than 24 hours when possible.

The specimen is collected on an ordinary cotton wool sterile swab, the patient being told to stir this round in the fæces without outside contamination.

An emulsion of this is made in normal saline and plated in the usual way.

Neutral-red bile salt peptone lactose agar is the medium which we mostly use, but if failure to obtain abnormal organisms on this occurs malachite green or brilliant green media may be tried. These latter media will sometimes grow an organism which fails to appear on the former, but it must be remembered that they are incapable of growing many of the varieties and so it is well always to continue plating on the first named during any repeated trials.

In a large majority of cases non-lactose-fermenting bacilli are obtained at the first test, sometimes however, two, and more rarely a large number of examinations are necessary: but it is our own experience that it is of the utmost rarity completely to fail to find these bacilli, though we have had to examine as many as 25 specimens.

A colony which is non-lactose fermenting should be cultured for the vaccine. They may vary from one, to several hundreds in proportion to those of the bacillus coli ; or they may be as many as one hundred per cent. of the colonies obtained ; also they vary considerably in the same case at different times.

It is comparatively rare, (only in about one per cent. of all cases), to find more than one type of abnormal bacillus in the same patient: if this does occur, it is necessary to add both varieties to the vaccine.

Cultures are made from these abnormal colonies on agar slopes. It appears better not to allow any undue cooling in this process and the slopes should have been previously warmed in the incubator.

These are incubated at 37 degrees Centigrade for 16 hours, this time giving the best results, and cultures should be washed up with as little delay as possible after this time.

If the growth is of the average size one slope is used, if decidedly feeble, two or even three may be necessary and if prolific half a slope should be used.

This culture or cultures are washed up in about 6 cc. of normal sterile saline, the tube sealed and the culture killed by immersion in water heated to 60 degrees centigrade for one hour.

The emulsion is then put into a bottle and normal saline added to bring it up to 25 cc. and .25 cc. (which is equivalent to one per cent.) of the following antiseptic mixture added :—

Distilled Lysol   .. 1 part
Absolute alchol   .. 3 parts

The doses of this vaccine used are as follows :—

No. 1   ..   ..   .. .04
No. 2   ..   ..   .. .08
No. 3 2
No. 4 4
No. 5 6
No. 6 9

If the injection of any dose causes a marked local tenderness, lasting more than four days or a general reaction which seriously incapacitates the patient, the next dose given, after a suitable interval, should not be larger but identical in quantity with the one which has aroused the reaction.

If no reaction of any kind follows the dose then the next one of the series can be omitted and the next but one administered. As much as 2 c.c. may finally be given: we have never found it necessary to exceed this dose.

In the body of this book will be found repeated exhortations as to the spacing out of the doses. If a favourable response is obtained, no second dose should be given as long as improvement continues and great care is needed not to mistake a slight and temporary setback for such a definite cessation of benefit as warrants a further injection.

As an antiseptic we much prefer Lysol to Carbolic, as the local reaction is less and the value of the vaccine is longer maintained in its full virulence.

If two organisms are present in a patient the usual quantity of each may be added to the vaccine without altering the dosage stated.

Polyvalent Vaccine.

For this purpose we divide the bacilli into three groups and make a Polyvalent Vaccine of each type.

Class 1. Those producing acid in glucose no fermentation with lactose or saccharose.

Class 2. Producing acid and gas in glucose, nothing in lactose or saccharose.

Class 3. Giving acid and gas in glucose and saccharose and nothing in lactose.

Day by day as abnormal organisms are grown, they should be washed up and killed without waiting for the result of the sugar reactions which determine their nature.

It is advisable to do this in the least amount of saline necessary so as to reduce the bulk of the stock. When the group of the organisms has been decided according to their sugar reaction, stock bottles of about

400 c.c. capacity are prepared and the killed cultures added to their respective bottles until about two hundred cases have been included of each type.

The total number of slopes added should be accurately known so that from this and the capacity of the bottle the strength of the stock can be estimated. An amount of antiseptic is added from time to time according to the bulk of the stock. For actual use sufficient is withdrawn to represent the quantity of one slope, (this amount usually being about 1.5 to 2 c.c.), and this is added to a bottle containing 22 c.c. of normal saline and the usual preservatives added.

The dose of this final vaccine will correspond to that described for the autogenous preparation.

APPENDIX C.

Analysis of Cases.

IT will be perhaps of some interest to give a more detailed analysis of the 500 cases which form the clinical record cited in the body of this book. We classify them in regard to results as A B C and D. A are the excellent and rather remarkable results, B the thoroughly good results, C the moderate and more disappointing ones and D the failures.

		A.	B.	C.	D.
11	Chronic Skin Disease		6	4	1
	(Eczema (2) Psoriasis (3) Acne (2) Urticaria (2), Erythema Nodosum (2).				
27	Anæmia	2	19	6	
5	Bacilluria	2	2	1	
43	Chronic Rheumatism	7	32	3	1
6	Gout		3	3	
3	Lumbago	1	2		
1	Fibrositis				1
77	Rheumatoid Arthritis	9	29	31	8
16	Sciatica	5	6	5	
6	Neuritis	2	2	2	

		A.	B.	C.	D.
12	Epilepsy		8	3	1
33	Chronic Headache	6	15	10	2
87	Neurasthenia	11	54	19	3
5	Hysteria		2	3	
3	Insomnia	1	2		
7	Mania	1	4	1	1
7	Graves disease		7		
10	General Debility		9	1	
2	Hyperpiesis	1	1		
1	Alcoholism		1		
17	Chronic Gastritis	5	10	1	1
38	Chronic Colitis	6	18	13	1
3	Constipation		1	2	
5	Cholecystitis		4	1	
12	Chronic Catarrh of upper air passages	2	7	3	
9	Asthma		7	2	
3	Chronic Bronchitis		3		
1	Emphysema				1
32	Malignant disease		20	9	3

The chapter on Malignant Disease gives the more extended survey of the last cases and it has to be realized fully how desperate they all were before a true estimate of results can be attained. There are several that might almost have been classed in Division A. for speed and effectiveness of response, but as we have not yet been able to observe many cancer cases for very long

periods of time, it is better to make only
the more modest claim. There can be as
yet no claim to have cured any one of them.
A number have died : but as no one of them
when undertaken had an expectation of
life of more than a few weeks and as nearly
all were in severe pain necessitating constant administration of morphia, we have
taken relief of pain, prolongation of life and
restored sense of well-being as the factors
by which to classify the cases. It is interesting that in several cases there has
been quite a long period (8—12 months)
of enjoyable life instead of misery and then
a mercifully sudden death.

We have notes of seven cases of Chronic
Tuberculosis. They can be classed as 3A
and 4B. But the warning given in the
text must be repeated that the value of
intestinal vaccine treatment in these and
similar cases, is to clear up the states that
have become very chronic and notably
improve general health. Whenever Tuber-

culosis is active, the utmost care is needed
lest an aggravation ensure ; but when a
case is partially arrested it is possible by our
vaccines to turn partial into more complete
arrest.

The balance of our 500 cases comprises
a handful of Chronic diseases, too few in
numbers for any analysis to be of value.
A disseminated Sclerosis, for instance, did
well (Class B), but this disease is notoriously
subject to remissions.   One case of Lymph-
adenoma   seemed   to   respond   (Class   B)
but no conclusion can be drawn from one
case.   We have referred in the text to the
two Glycosuria cases and to one case of
optic neuritis.   We have two in our list :
both   did   well,   one   was   almost   certainly
toxic in origin and of the other it is difficult
to speak with certainty as to the cause.   We
have had only one Dysmenorrhœa to treat,
with a very satisfactory result, but we cannot
help thinking that this is a class of case which
should   prove   amenable   to   these   vaccines.

INDEX.

i.

iv.

www.ingramcontent.com/pod-product-compliance
Lightning Source LLC
Chambersburg PA
CBHW030555270326
41927CB00007B/936